HOW A SEIZURE SAVED MY LIFE

Janet Lee Glaser

books and novels
by Janet Glaser
(available on Amazon.com)

I'll do it My Myself

The Invisible Mask

The Surrogate Mother

The Domino Effect

The Heart of a Clown
(an autobiography

Madison's Ideal

Escape from Truth-N-Love

Stop Light Short Stories

(coming soon)

Make Believe Love

Born Different

SPECIAL THANKS TO:

My husband, Larry, my children, Sandy, Keith, John and Kelli for their prayers and help, Dr. Christopher Bradley, Dr. Stephen Reitman, Neurosurgeon Dr. Hertzel Soumekh, Grossmont Hospital in San Diego, California and the many friends who prayed, brought in food and flowers. Thanks also to Ralph Erwin, my editor. Without all of you I would have not made it. <u>Most of all, I thank the Lord</u> for being with me every step of the way.

This is a true story of how a seizure helped doctors discover two dangerous brain aneurysms and repair them before major disaster occurred in my life. The purpose of this little booklet is to encourage and bless anyone going through hard times.

Published by
JayJay Books
9500 Harritt Road
Suite 193
Lakeside, CA 92040

HOW A SEIZURE SAVED MY LIFE

I don't remember much about Saturday, January 6, 2006, but my husband, Larry, tells me we were eating and I suddenly stared into space. When he asked if I was all right, I didn't respond and when he asked a second time, I still didn't reply. I do remember stirring food, but I don't remember fixing dinner. I wasn't in pain. I was just confused. After we finished eating, I sat on the couch. My heart pounded. My back started hurting and I was sweating. Larry called 911. When the paramedics arrived, I could hear their questions, but I couldn't respond. "What is your name?

How much do you weight? Who
is the president?"

They took me to the
hospital and ran a CT Scan and
an M.R.I. The result: two
aneurysms in my brain behind
my right eye, but no explanation
for the seizure activity leading to
the test results. The doctor
explained, "An aneurysm is a
balloon-like bulge in the wall of
a brain artery. If the bulge tears
and bleeds, nearby cells can be
damaged. It usually happens in
an artery wall that is weak or
defective. If it ruptures, blood
running into the brain can cause a
stroke or death."

Aneurysm! The word
petrified me because my

husband's best friend died from a ruptured aneurysm at the age of 38.

Neurologist   Dr. Christopher Bradley told me the seizure was not caused by the aneurysm. In fact, he wasn't sure why it happened, but ordered some tests. He said it could have been the result of a past head injury.

Neurosurgeon, Dr. Hertzel Soumekh informed me there was good and bad news. The good news was the aneurysms had not ruptured. The bad news was there was a 50% chance they would hemorrhage and, if that happened, there would be a 70% chance I would either be an invalid the rest of my life, or die.

The doctor said there are two ways to treat brain aneurysms.

Endovascular procedures are done in x-ray labs by specially-trained doctors who guide catheters through arteries from the groin to the brain. Platinum coils that create blood clots are then released into the aneurysms to create blood clots that prevents rupturing. The doctor told me one of my aneurysms could be treated this way, but the other one was larger and would require the more invasive open surgery.

In the open surgery procedure, part of my skull bone would be cut away so the surgeon could put a clip where the artery was bulging. That would prevent blood from entering my brain and causing further damage. Both doctors felt I was not a candidate for the Endovascular procedure, but it was my choice. Since I had no bleeding or serious symptoms, I could take my chances and not have the surgery, but, if the aneurysms would rupture, I would be in serious trouble.

After consulting my family, I told them I did not want to live the rest of my life fearing a ruptured aneurysm or becoming a constant worry to my loving husband, four children and seven grandchildren.

Therefore, my surgery was scheduled for January 17, 2006. The doctor told me the surgery would take about six hours and my stay in intensive care most likely would be five to seven days.

Dr. Soumekh tried to relieve my anxiety by asking, "How do you want your hair cut?"

I laughed feeling like I was going to a beautician. He smiled and continued, "I can either shave all your hair and it will grow back at the same time, or shave it three inches back from your forehead. That way you will have hair and you can wear those head bands that are so popular until the hair grows back."

I decided to have 'my hair cut' three inches in the front and my family purchased every color head band so I had one to match every outfit I owned. I still laugh when I remember, even though the doctor looked like he had no sense of humor, he really did. He also told me he was going to give me a free face lift. Free, along with the brain surgery.

Was I scared? You bet! Knowing I could not face this ordeal alone, I called several people and asked them to pray for me. The word spread and I soon had many people praying for me, some I didn't even know. Thanks to God and to my praying friends, it worked!   I firmly believe I would not be here today if these 'angels" and my loving family had not said a lot of prayers for me.

The prayers of my husband, Larry, sons, John and Keith, my daughters, Sandy and Kelli and a few close friends gave me a wonderful sense of peace as they rolled me into the operating room.

The doctor thought I was asleep, but I heard him say, "There are no guarantees in this operation. I must tell you, she might not make it or she could be paralyzed, but I'm not going to let that happen."

The doctor left and soon someone rolled my bed into surgery. I opened my eyes as Larry held my ands and the children walked along beside my bed and said, "I feel so peaceful." And, I really did.

Eight hours later, my family and friends greeted me in the intensive care unit.

I don't remember much after the surgery. I remember saying, "Well, they put my brain back the right way," when they rolled me back into my room. My son, John, later revealed to me how important it was to him that I still had my sense of humor. It gave him the peace of mind he needed.

The days were spent sleeping and eating. I wasn't aware of having a room mate or
what went on around me. I wasn't in pain and I didn't know what I looked like. A friend from church brought in a camera and took a picture of me. I wondered why she did that. Later, when I saw the picture, I was horrified. Both my eyes were black, I had a bruise on my right chin. Now when I look at the picture, I see where God brought me from and thank Him for where I am today. She did me a favor without realizing it.

I don't remember who came to see me, but I knew many came because I had lots of flowers and cards. Every time I woke up I saw my husband and children in the room. One day they took me for a spinal tap. when I returned, I had to lay flat on my back for several hours. Right after they put me in bed, a woman brought in my dinner. I was awake and felt okay. I looked at the tray on my chest and thought of me eating while lying down. "How am I going to eat?" I asked Kelli and John. "We'll feed you," John said. He went to my right and Kelli was on my left. Kelli put a towel around my neck and they took turns feeding me. She was so funny, I couldn't help but laugh. "Open your mouth, Mommy," she said as she held the spoon to my mouth. I felt like a baby. I was so weak I had trouble chewing. "Chew your food, Mommy," she said and smiled at me. John would give me a bite and wipe my mouth, then Kelli would give me another bite. They were so sweet and caring. I still smile as I remember my two grown children feeding me.

Though I had been told I would be in intensive care five to seven days, I was there only two days. The operation was on Tuesday and I went home Saturday. All the specialists involved were amazed at my rapid recovery.

The doctor said I had survived one of the 'most serious of serious surgeries' with no ill effects and, I am thrilled to say, I can still play the piano, read, write and do other normal things just as I could before this happened.

Several weeks later I went to the doctor to have the staples removed. The incision had been made from ear to ear along my hairline. I looked like the mother of Frankenstein with my hair shaved three inches back and staples holding my skin together. I was happy to have the head bands and many people complemented me when I wore them. Anyway, when the doctor removed the staples, his sense of humor, if you call it that, surfaced.   He had used forty staples. I expected it to hurt when he removed them, but it was just a little sting. I felt happy to get them out as they were starting to itch and pull. Each one he removed, he put in a small box. When he finished he asked my daughter if she wanted to keep them as a souvenir. She said no. Next he asked my son and he too, said no. Finally he asked me. I laughed and said, "No. recycle them." Everyone laughed at the thought of recycling staples. I suppose some people would have saved them, but I didn't want those as a memory.

I did have challenging recovery symptoms, such as tightness in my head, electric-like currents "racing" though my head and face, headaches, "itching" in my brain, changes in taste and smell senses, and fatigue. I couldn't tolerate vibrations or loud noise like a lot of people talking or music with a heavy drum beat or base. It made my brain feel like someone put marbles in a box and was shaking them around. I had a hard time staying in church when the music was playing because I bothered me so much. Traveling was difficult because of vibrations of the car. I found some relief from the symptoms with the use of ice packs. At night, a warm bath while listening to nature sounds behind piano music helped my brain to relax and I slept better. I took medicine and I became an "expert" at resting. The recovery was a long time and I became impatient, but I knew God was in control.

There remains the mystery of the seizure. What caused it? Dr. Bradley said I had epilepsy, that I probably had small seizures often, but wasn't aware of them. I didn't remember ever having one.

I think I know the reason. God "gave" me the seizure to prevent a fatal aneurysm and make me more grateful than ever for the many blessings I enjoy each day.

The Boat Trip

(The Lord gave gave me this story one night during my recovery from the brain surgery.)

I knew the trip could be rough, but I didn't realize how difficult it would be. I got into the small boat and felt alone. The river bubbled around the boat making waves, so I held on while I walked to my seat in the rear of the craft. The rocking made me feel dizzy, but I said, "I can do this. I can do this."

I sat down, closed my eyes and tried to relax. Then I heard someone get on the boat with me and I opened my eyes. He was tall, had sparkling eyes and a tender smile. "I'm your guide.

Just sit back and relax. I know this river. I know the rapids and I know where the large rocks are. I'll get you there safely. You don't have to do anything," he said.

That would be difficult for me because I did everything myself. I was strong and didn't need any help. I wasn't a baby. I looked dubiously at the stranger and asked, "What is your name?"

"You know me. I've known you since you were born. Don't you remember?"

I closed my eyes and tried to think who knew me all my life, but no one came to my mind.

My guide untied the boat from the shoring, sat down, started the engine and guided us to the center of the river. The boat started rocking harder and harder, then it went into a circle of water. My heart pounded. I grabbed an oar to help get us out of the whirl pool, but the guide leaned over, took the oar from me, and said, "Remember, I'll take care of everything. I know the river."

I hesitantly let go of the oar and held onto the side of my chair. "Who are you?" I asked again.

He smiled gently and replied, "Keep thinking. Soon you'll remember."

The river became more swift and water splashed into the boat. I saw rapids of white water a few feet ahead, and screamed.

"We're going to die. Take me back! Let me out!"

"Don't worry, I know these rapids," he said. "It will be rough, but come sit close to me and I'll keep you safe. I'm going through the rapids with you."

He took my hand, helped me sit next to him, put his left arm around me and steered the boat with his right hand. I felt the tenderness of his embrace and a love I could not understand. The boat started floundering in the rapid water. "Let me go," I cried. "Let me go or we'll both drown."

"No, I can't let you go. I love you and I won't let you go. I will always be with you where ever you go."

"I don't understand. Why do we have to go through the rapids? Why can't we take a different route? There has to be a better way."

"This is the only way. I'm sorry the trip is so rough, but remember, I'm going with you."

The boat tossed and filled with cold water. I hit my arm on the railing and tears filled my eyes.

He held me closer and when I looked into his face, I saw tears in his eyes. "I'm sorry you have to go through all this, but, but . . ."

Larger rapids loomed ahead of the boat. I held tightly to his arm and closed my eyes. The boat tossed and turned in circles.

We hit a large rock and plumped sideways almost turning over. He held me tighter.

The rapids became less rough before he spoke again. "I'm so sorry you had to go through that," he said again. He removed his arm from around me and wiped his eyes with the back of his hand. "I wish you didn't have to go through it."

I wiped my tears, looked into his gentle face, and asked, "What is the name of this river?"

He smiled and said, "The Life River."

Suddenly I recognized him. It was Jesus guiding me through the rough times, putting his arms around me in troubled waters, and crying with me. It was Jesus who was guiding me along life's brutal river. It was Jesus who cried with me and knew my fears.

I looked to the side and saw many small boats capsized along the shore. "What are those boats doing there?" I asked.

His mouth set in a straight line and wrinkles creased his forehead. "Those are the people who refused to let me go with them because they thought they knew the way by themselves. It makes me sad to see them, but they refused my help."

The rapids stopped and we were floating on a placid blue lake surrounded by tall pine trees. Small fluffy white clouds floated in the bright blue sky.

The warm sun penetrated my wet clothes as I looked at Jesus. "Thank you," I said as tears slid out of my eyes.

He guided the boat to a beach, took my hand and helped me out onto the soft white sand. I looked at him and said, "I love you."

"I love you, too. I have always loved you. I have to leave you for just a little while, but I'm asking someone else to stay with you until I return. Everything you need or want is here."

"Where are you going?"

"I have to get another person through the rapids of the River of Life. I'll be back soon. Maybe you can help the other person because you both took the same journey. I'll leave a letter with you so if you get lonely, you can read it."

I watched him walk back to the boat and pull away, but I knew He would be back. I opened the letter and read, "I will never leave you or forsake you."

I sat on the sand, closed my eyes, felt the warm breeze in my hair and cried. I felt warm arms around me and opened my eyes, but saw no one. I knew, however, someone was with me and I felt peaceful and happy.

POSTSCRIPT

When I became a Christian, I thought life would be easy, that I would have no troubles, but I was wrong. I walked through the storm of abuse as a child and Jesus walked and cried with me. God gave everyone the gift of choice. Choices people make affect others in a positive or negative way. He promised us the roses, but we also have to take the thorns.

I wrote this little booklet as a testimony of God's grace and love. He brought me through childhood problems and the most serious of serious surgeries. I know He walked with me. I made a choice of taking His hand as he leads me through the troubles of this life, knowing there is a peaceful beautiful place waiting for me in heaven. I can see the rose, as I walk through the thorns of life.

I wish could say I'm back to my normal self, but I'm not. I still have periodic headaches and have to rest more than I like. I don't have the drive I had earlier to go and do everything, but that could be because as I write this, I am 74 -years - old. Sometimes, when I feel bad, I get depressed. It's then, I praise Jesus for being with me and bringing me through the rapids of the Lake of Life. I live one day at a time and decided I will never let go of His hand, or try to take the boat oars because my guide, Jesus, knows the rapids on the River of Life. I wake up thanking Jesus for another day and asking Him to direct me. I also ask Him to help me follow His directions and not try to go my way.

Brain surgery wasn't easy, but many things in life are not easy. Without Jesus, I know I would not be alive or as healthy as I am. I am looking forward to the day when I see Him face to face, but until that day I resolve to enjoy each day with my children, grand children and great grand children. I praise God for His loving presence and how much He has done for me and I pray you will receive a blessing by reading this.

No one is perfect. All my life I pretended my life was perfect, but in 1987 reality loomed its head and the truth that I was an abused child became a reality.

(You may read more about this in my autobiography, *The Heart of a Clown* that can be purchased on Amazon.com. or Target.com.)

During my lowest times the Lord was with me and kept me from falling into the depths of total despair. The memories of how the Lord helped me through those hard times strengthened me when I had the brain surgery.

As in the Chinese belief of Yin and Yang (opposites), I

became a stronger Christian because of the dark side of life. The dark side makes the light that much brighter.

The Lord gave me many poems that helped me make it though the dankest hours of my life and reflect my intermost thoughts.

For a while, after the surgery, I though I lost the creative ability to write. I prayed and asked God not to take it away and He answered in a marvelous way. I have written and published several Christian novels and continue to work on others.

May the poems give you hope as you walk through your storms. <u>God is so merciful</u>.

A NEW DAY

THIS IS A NEW TIME
GOD GAVE TODAY;
A BLANK PAGE TO FOLLOW
IN HIS WAY.
A DAY TO CHOOSE GOOD,
OVER THE BAD,
A DAY TO BE HAPPY
AND NOT FEEL SAD.
THIS DAY IS MINE,
GOD GAVE IT TO ME.
GOD HELP ME TO BE
WHAT YOU WANT
ME TO BE.

NO PLACE ELSE

*THERE'S NO PLACE ELSE
I'D RATHER BE
THAN HAVE YOU SITTING
CLOSE TO ME.
THERE'S NOTHING ELSE I'D
RATHER DO
THAN BEING RIGHT HERE
NEXT TO YOU.
THERE'S NO ONE ELSE
THAT I KNOW
WHO KNOWS ME WELL, YET
LOVES ME SO,
SO MUCH LOVE I CAN'T
BELIEVE
YOU EVEN CRY WHEN I
GRIEVE.
THANK YOU FOR THE LOVE
YOU SHARE ALL AROUND
ME, EVERYWHERE.*

TODAY I CHOOSE
_TO_
REMEMBER
THE GOOD, NOT
THE BAD.
REMEMBER
THE HAPPY, NOT
THE SAD.
REMEMBER
THE SUNSHINE,
NOT THE RAIN.
REMEMBER
THE JOY,
NOT THE PAIN.
REMEMBER
THE PEACE,
NOT THE FEAR,
AND ALWAYS REMEMBER,
GOD IS NEAR

COUNT YOUR BLESSINGS

*SOMETIMES MY LIFE GETS
WEARY.
I THINK I HAVE NO FRIEND.
I GO THROUGH THAT DARK
TUNNEL WHICH SEEMS TO
HAVE NO END.
SOMETIMES I AM LONELY
AND CLOUDS COVER THE
SUN,
FOR ALL I SEE IS SADNESS
AND LIFE IS NO MORE FUN.
I KEEP MY EYES ON JESUS
AND TRUSTING IN THE
LORD.
AT THE END OF THE
TUNNEL THERE IS A GREAT
REWARD.
FOR GOD WILL NOT
FORSAKE ME IN TIMES OF*

DEEP DESPAIR. HIS ARMS
REACH OUT TOWARD ME
AND HE IS ALWAYS THERE.
JUST LOOK BEYOND THAT
TUNNEL.
THERE IS A LIGHT THAT
SHINES.
FOR JESUS CHRIST IS
SAYING,
"JUST PUT YOUR HAND IN
MINE."

MORE GOOD THAN BAD

*THERE ARE TIMES WHEN
THINGS GO WRONG AND
TRIALS ARE AROUND.
AT THOSE TIMES YOU'D
LIKE TO PUT YOUR
TROUBLES UNDERGROUND.
AT THE TIME WHEN YOU'RE
DEPRESSED AND DON'T
KNOW WHERE TO TURN,
MAKE A LIST BOTH GOOD
AND BAD AND VERY SOON
YOU'LL LEARN
GOD HAS GIVEN MUCH
MORE GOOD. THE BAD IS
MUCH, MUCH LESS.
THANK THE LORD FOR ALL
HE'S DONE. DON'T DWELL*

Janet Glaser

ON YOUR DISTRESS.
IN A MOMENT YOU WILL
FIND DEPRESSION
DISAPPEARS.
THE LORD WILL GIVE YOU
PEACE OF MIND AND SOON
A SMILE APPEARS.

NOTE:

This little booklet was written to encourage and hopefully make you feel closer to our Lord and Savior, knowing He will help you through all your problems if you ask and let Him. May God bless you. For more copies, contact

Janet Glaser
Janover60@sbcglobal.net
or
619-825-0240